Natural Remedies With Herbs And Spices

Helen Mayhew

About This Book

This book takes the myth and magic out of complementary medicine and presents us with a simple, straightforward formula for helping ourselves to better health. For far too long, the alternative to drug-based medicine was to take another medicine labelled 'natural' or 'alternative'.
Usually rather expensive and provided without the confidence installed by the backing of a practitioner. Now the gap between the two has been bridged by this straightforward down-to earth advice on integrating natural remedies into our day-to-day living via the Spice Shelf. This little fountain of knowledge, liberally illustrated with delightful live drawings by the author, and containing as it does such a wealth of invaluable information ranging from the treatments of acne to wounds, the making of cookies to combat the effects of junk food. Several different cost effective and pleasant ways of relieving that bane of society - stress etc. It should be on the spice shelf of every home in the country (that is when it is not being pored over, laughed with and thoroughly enjoyed by its readers).
Containing as it does something to help people in every age range, it can be given as a very useful present to suit all

occasions and I am sure will prove to be a real treasure to its readers for years to come.

The medical information and advice in this book are based upon the experience ad research of the author. Persons using this book should consult an appropriate health care provider when questions of medical treatment and care arise. The author assumes no responsibility and is not liable for adverse effects resulting from the use of any advice or information contained in this book.

No part of this publication may be reproduced or transmitted in any form or by any means, electronic or mechanical, including photocopy,
recording, or any information storage and retrieval system not known or to be invented, without permission in writing from the publisher, except by a reviewer who wishes to quote brief passages in connection with a review written for inclusion in a magazine, newspaper, or broadcast.

CONTENTS

Introduction	9
Allspice	14
Angleica	16
Aniseed	19
Basil	23
Bayleaf	25
Caraway	28
Cayenne pepper	30
Celery	33
Chervil & Chives	35
Cinnamon	36
Cloves	40
Coriander & Cumin	42
Dill	43
Fennel	45

Garlic	48
Ginger	51
MACE	55
Marjoram	57
Mint	60
Mustard	67
Nutmeg	69
Parsley	71
Pepper	74
Rosemary	76
Saffron	81
Sage	82
Tarragon	86
Thyme	87

Introduction

All of us use herbs and spices in one form or another in our day-to- day cooking, whether it be only mint sauce to be served with roast lamb or the more adventurous mixtures when trying out exotic foreign dishes.

The spice rack is one of the most under-appreciated and underused pieces of equipment in our kitchens, yet it is one of the safest, cheapest and most readily available medicine chests which no home should be without.

Everyone, from the busy career person with a cold coming just when they have a deadline to meet, the frantic housewife with a child who has suffered a nasty fall just when the doctor, chemist and shops are shut, the menopause sufferer who does not wish to 'bother' a busy GP, yet feels at the end of her tether, the elderly with aching joints who, having been told that they just 'have to live with it' feel that they just cannot, can find some relief using the herbs and spices which they probably already have in their homes, and if not, can be purchased inexpensively in their local stores.

No longer do we have to fill a first-aid cupboard with a mixture of proprietary drugs which we may or may not need before their sell-by date has expired, making it necessary to throw them out and buy more. Instead we will help ourselves to health in a safe, pleasant and tasty way.

Remembering always that self-diagnosis without expert training and experience is IMPOSSIBLE, self-help is readily available.

This little book, hopefully, will show YOU how.

My first remembrance of healing in the home is an incident which occurred when I was very young. Having been scratched rather badly by my pet kitten 'Chuckles' (no doubt in self-defence against being squeezed to death in the ecstasy of the moment!) I was scooped up by my grandmamma who promptly sucked the dirt out of my scratch, spat the viscous fluid onto the ground, then proceeded to lick the wound while telling me that 'a lady's spittle is the most antiseptic thing on earth and that is why mother animals lick their babies to clean them and to kill all their bad germs'. This was VERY confusing to me as at that tender age I thought that spitting was only done by road menders, night-watchmen and the rag-and-bone man when he talked about 'him over the water', yet here was my lady grandmamma spitting away like a builders navvy ... also ... if licking was the best way to kill germs why did my mama always use that dreadful soapy sponge on my face when I was contentedly licking honey off my mouth at supper time?

Puzzled I may have been, but my scratch was not only forgotten but healed without any further treatment or trouble, even though the incident had occurred on our back lawn/kitchen-garden which would have sent many mothers today screaming for the disinfectant, ointment, plasters etc, then worrying for the next few days as to whether sepsis would occur. .. or worse! Many children suffered lock-jaw from similar everyday wounds ... but they did not have a grandmamma like mine!

Through the years of the Second World War, I do not remember our family ever having to call our doctor away from his important work, yet, living as we did in the centre of Plymouth, we often experienced happenings which could have merited his healing presence. . . not least being made homeless on more than one occasion by bombs seeming to make a habit of destroying our homes (probably due to the fact that my family chose to live by the Naval Dockyard, the railway station and the city centre and refusing stoically to 'run away to the country'). We shared a series of cold-water flats, rooms, garages and derelict buses with people from all walks of life, some of whom travelled with their own personal vermin which most of us would shudder away from today, but which provided wonderful entertainment for young children confined for long hours in an air-raid shelter! My mother had to be ever watchful in my case as I loved everybody, including the old lady in the back room with her endless supply of fleas of many different hues which obligingly jumped onto me if I put my hands near enough to them, and the horse belonging to the rag-and-bone man which would rub its scabby nose on my face as I hugged its knees and pulled its tail! I spent a great deal of my early childhood in a tin bath in front of the fire being almost poached in tansy tea to avoid becoming as vermin-infested as my everyday associates! Had mother or grandmamma known that I was also privileged to handle pet mice and cockroaches, I would have been washed away!

Being an inquisitive child, I also spent a lot of time with my mother in the air-raid shelters and in the various 'safe' places where she and the other women of the district would gather to exchange news about the most recent happenings and which weed, herb or food they had used to 'pep themselves up'. It was often very confusing for me to understand why, for instance, the same cabbage which could stop an old person's knees from aching if it was rubbed on them, would also make my hair nice and curly if I ate the dreadful stuff!

However, I obtained an invaluable grounding in home healing which was to pave the way for my interest in medicine, (both the orthodox and alternatives types) and lead to my becoming a doctor in the latter, with my paths travelling all over the world in search of new and unusual, yet simple medicines.

Throughout teenage and young adulthood, my mother and stepfather saw to it that my academic and scientific learning about medicine was rich and full, including as it did, orthodox, homoeopathic and herbal training ... while maturity brought me back into contact with my own father who is one of those special breed of people known as the 'wise ones' in his locality and from him I learned to dovetail all the little snippets from early childhood into their correct places. Parenthood with its attendant worries over the health of my children in an increasingly unhealthy environment really tested my knowledge to the full, and, I am happy to say that my family are all in the best of health and spirits using home remedies. This little book has come into being due to the constant urging by patients, colleagues, friends and neighbours to set this knowledge down in easily understandable form in handy-sized books which can be kept in kitchen, medicine cupboard or pocket, needing only a quick glance in an emergency in order to offer fast and effective first-aid in the home, without either having to call a busy doctor or rush out to buy preparatory drugs, be they synthetic or 'natural'.

In the case of serious illness or injury, it is always wise to consult your family doctor and to abide by his decision regarding the correct course of treatment. However, more and more general practitioners are embracing some of the so-called 'alternative' forms of treatment and are usually pleased to advise patients regarding forms of self-help.

One more reason for using the remedies which I have suggested is the fact that while one may have the faintest reservations regarding the safety in use of their intended medication, that fear prevents the body from accepting and making full use of that medication. . . however. . . if that medicine is home-made from everyday foodstuffs, what is there to fear? As all of the ingredients of good health (and indeed for ill health also) are to be found in our diet and lifestyle, it is very simple to bring about changes for the better in these, PROVIDED that we are taught how to use them to our best advantage ... I hope that this small offering of mine will be of some use in setting your feet on the road to self-help and self-improvement using the healers in your home.

Allspice

How very appropriate that a book about spices should start with that very versatile and all-embracing taste experience, Allspice having as it does, a flavour of clove, cinnamon, ginger and pepper, hence its very suitable name.

Allspice is actually the fruit of the pimento or Jamaica pepper and its penetrating warmth will stimulate the gastro-intestinal tract if taken internally, while an external application brings relief to muscular pain.

A very good gripe-water can be quickly and inexpensively made by adding 2 teaspoons of Allspice berries to half a litre of wine vinegar or cider vinegar, shaking well and keeping tightly stoppered in the refrigerator. For cases of colic, flatulence or griping stomach pains, shake bottle well, allow to settle then add 1 teaspoonful of Allspice vinegar to a cup of hot water and sip slowly ... relief is not long in coming.

To ease muscular pain, a very warming and pleasant smelling ointment can be made by adding 1 teaspoon of powdered Allspice to 4 oz or 125 gm of pure vegetable lard and cooking in a covered glass dish at a low temperature for half an hour, then pouring into a warmed glass jar and waiting until it is cool before covering... keep In the refrigerator to remind you that it is available at all times, as it is invaluable for ease of cramp, neurasthenia (pains which occur when the nerves are in need of stimulation or relaxation), neuralgia and rheumatism.

Angleica

What a pretty name is Angelica, and just as it conjures up sweet thoughts, so too the herb itself is sweet to take. For this reason, it is a boon to harassed mothers of small children as, although medicine is often refused by the sick child who needs it, the sweet concoction of Angelica is not only taken without demur but even welcomed!

A good remedy for colds, colic, coughs, pleurisy, respiratory disorders, rheumatism, indigestion and urinary disorders, it is certainly one of the most important remedies on the shelf.
Add 1 teaspoon of chopped Angelica to 1 miniature bottle of brandy and keep in the refrigerator. .. this will keep for years if not needed, so is a very good method of making sure that you always have some to hand in an emergency. Use in the following manner:
For children's colic and windy pains, add 5 drops of the mixture to 1 teaspoon of honey and give to drink in warm water. For adult indigestion, add 10 drops to 1 tablespoon of hot water and sip slowly.
For chills, fevers, influenza etc., add 1 tablespoon to 1 tablespoon of cider vinegar or lemon juice in 1 cupful of very hot water sweetened with honey if required, and drink HOT.

This Angelica brandy makes a very pleasant digest if liqueur which can be a very welcome Christmas or birthday present, especially for digestive or chest complaint sufferers.

Another very good standby to make for your store cupboard is a pot of Angelica honey which is simply made by finely chopping 1 oz or 25 gm of Angelica and stirring it into a 1 lb of clear honey ... this will also keep indefinitely ... if out of reach! For bronchitis, coughs, croup, chronic sore throats or tonsillitis, insomnia, pleurisy, pains in the joints caused by extension and flatulence, take 1 teaspoon each night and morning also when the symptoms are most severe ... beware of children being able to reach this most delightful of medicines, or you may find that you have an empty pot just when it is most needed (this I found out to my cost many years ago!)

For pain caused by gout, arthritis, rheumatism and cystitis, a tea made by adding 1 teaspoon of seeds, leaves or stems of the Angelica plant added to boiling water bring great relief.

If flannels or similar cloths are soaked in this mixture while it is as hot as the hands can bear, then wrung out and applied immediately to congested chests and painful joints, these poultices quickly bring relief from pain and swelling. This Angelica tea, if drunk regularly, is reputed to 'bless the drinker with a disgust for an excess of spiritful liquors'!

To my mind, the most wonderful property of Angelica is its taste, which is so pleasant that, should you be caught unawares and not have anything prepared, you can simply give the sufferer a piece of candied Angelica to suck and the benefit will very soon be apparent.

If you are fortunate enough to have a piece of garden which you could use for growing this herb, you would find it a real boon.

Angelica is a large, aromatic plant which is a joy to behold, having as it does, downy triangular leaves and hollow stalks which bear umbels of frothy white and occasionally pale purple flowers, which lend themselves well to flower arrangements. Not being a believer in letting anything go to waste, I use every part of my plant to benefit good health, and so ward off ill health in my family.

The flower umbels, dipped in light batter and fried as 'fairy pancakes' make a tasty desert for children and one which also relaxes the intestinal tract after heavy meals or 'junk' foods.

The raw stalks are absolutely delicious when eaten with cream cheese, tasting, as they do, rather like sweet celery.

The roots can be boiled or braised and used in place of fennel as an unusual and piquant addition to a special meal, and the leaves are very tasty when eaten in mixed raw salads.

Any part of the herb can be chopped, added to boiling water, and used as a gargle for sore throats, a digestive tea for indigestion and heartburn, or a poultice for painful joints. Angelica is a truly versatile and wonderful herb, yet for me the best benefit of all is the fact that I can pop to my local shop and buy it already prepared and keep it ever handy in my larder or on the spice shelf.

Aniseed

Aniseed is a much overlooked herb in the kitchen which was prized in ancient Egypt and often used in Biblical times to pay taxes ... although it can no longer satisfy the taxman, it should still play a very important part in our lives as its main virtue is to aid our digestion and sweeten the breath.

In Virgil's time 'Mustace Cake' was given at the end of a marriage feast to prevent indigestion after the consumption of such a rich repast, hence our tradition today of ensuring that all guests have a piece of the wedding cake! Virgil must have had similar tastes to mine for I can well remember the spankings I had as a child for eating Aunt Boadicea's seedy-cake before it had had time to cool!

Simple indigestion can be relieved swiftly by chewing a few seeds, or prevented by adding a few seeds to the cooking, be it savoury or sweet. The addition of Aniseed when cooking cabbage or parsnips not only adds a piquancy which is quite delightful, but also gives the bonus that the juice, when strained off, yields a tasty, clear soup to start or finish the meal which actually helps all that has gone before, or is to come after, to digest in complete comfort ... what a godsend!

In stubborn cases, pour half a pint of boiling water on 1 teaspoon of bruised seeds, add 1 tablespoon of honey, stir well, chill and bottle ... keep refrigerated and take 1-3 teaspoons after each meal.

This mixture is also extremely effective for colic.

One of Aniseed's many virtues is that it is anti-spasmodic: it can be very useful to people who suffer from asthma and other complaints of a bronchitic nature.

In an emergency I have administered 1 teaspoon of crushed seeds
(I bashed them with a rolling-pin!) vigorously stirred in a teacupful of boiling water and trickle the mixture into the mouth of someone having a spasmodic asthma attack in the middle of the night; when no doctor was available and we lived in total seclusion without car, telephone or neighbours ... he not only lived to tell the tale, but now travels nowhere without his little pot of Aniseeds!

A mixture to keep in the refrigerator if one has children with dry coughs, asthma, bronchitis or catarrh can be made as follows:

Take 1 bottle of pure lemon juice, pour into a saucepan, add half a pound of clear honey and 1 oz of bruised Aniseeds. Bring to the boil stirring constantly, then simmer for 5 minutes. When this mixture is cold, it can be re bottled and used either in teaspoonful doses straight from the bottle, as a hot toddy last thing at night before retiring by adding 1 tablespoonful to a cup of hot water or, as a soothing chilled drink in cases of heat prostration, hiccoughs, epileptic attacks or abdominal migraine, by simply pouring a glass of iced water and adding a tablespoonful of the mixture and stirring well.

Aniseed can also be used as a very effective and pleasant mouthwash by simply adding crushed seeds to hot water. Elderly people, particularly those who are housebound, often suffer from dropsical conditions brought about by inactivity linked to inadequate nutrition and insufficient digestion, the three'I's which create most diseases prevalent today. Aniseed can be a great help here as, not only does it aid the digestion and ease flatulence - the fear of which often prevents elderly sufferers from eating as much as their bodies needs, it also is a sovereign remedy for the hiccoughs which so often accompany an otherwise much enjoyed meal. One very tasty way to 'take the medicine' is to put 1 heaped teaspoon of seeds into a boiling fowl, put into a much larger pan than is necessary, cover and boil in the usual way. The juices can be taken as hot broth, either between meals or, in the case of loss of appetite, in place of meals. The same can be done with any green or root vegetables to ensure that all of the nutrition is taken into the system without causing any bloating or discomfort.

Powdered Aniseed can be added to jams and jellies to make deliciously different desserts and, of course, it can still be taken in its original style ... in seed cakes which are welcomed by young and old alike.

Aniseed is one of the main ingredients of several liqueurs and aperitifs. A tasty and very different wine can be made by adding 1 oz of Aniseeds to any home-made wine during the fermentation stage ... absolutely delicious as a tonic!

Aniseed is a very useful herb to have on the spice shelf for another very important reason ... it is The Women's Wonderworker!

Dealing with the most common of female complaints, and one which generates the least sympathy from non-sufferers, is a very simple matter when one is a dedicated user of Aniseed ... I am of course referring to that scourge of womankind, painful periods!

To prevent the pains occurring, for three days before the start of a period do not drink any tea or coffee, but drink Aniseed tea made by putting 1 flat teaspoon of powdered seeds into a warmed earthenware pot and adding 1 litre of boiling water. Alternatively, put one pinch of powder or half a teaspoon of crushed seeds into a mug and pour on boiling water to fill. This tea should be drunk without milk, but can be sweetened with honey to taste if necessary.

As a compress for mastitis (swollen and inflamed or itching breasts) caused by either menses, milk-fever or the menopause, simply make tea as above, soak a cloth or flannel in the mixture, wring out and apply to the breasts as hot as can be borne without discomfort (on days when one is not expecting visitors and no travelling has to be done, these cloths can be worn inside an old brassiere and changed when necessary.) Oily skin is a complaint which cannot be understood or sympathised with by anyone who has not suffered from it. Sufferers take heart! Help is here with wonderful Aniseed! This tea, made as above, and drunk before retiring, also applied to the skin after washing, soon clears the problem ... wonderful!

Basil

Basil is a very wonderful spice herb in that it works very gently and thoroughly on the nervous system and, living as most of us do at a frantic pace almost guaranteed to put a strain on all but the strongest of systems, there are not many of us who would not benefit from its gentle and cheering action.

To a small bottle of almond, olive or sunflower oil add 1 teaspoon of dried Basil, keep in a warm place and shake daily ... I keep my bottle on the radiator shelf and it is always ready to hand if anyone needs it.

When feeling the need of Basil's ministrations, simply pour a little of the warm oil into the palm of your hand and sit quietly massaging your tensions away ... you will soon feel a new person as the relaxation steals through your system.

Basil oil makes an excellent application to massage into the muscles and ease the pains of wandering neuralgia, cramp and rheumatism, especially the dreadful night-cramps which only seem to strike when there is absolutely no medication in the house with this oil to hand, you need never fear that again, but . beware. . . this oil leaves you with a feeling of euphoria and sometimes it can be annoying to be full of the joys of spring when everyone else is trying to sleep!

It is very unusual to find a treatment that stimulates the nerves as most remedies only sedate, so Basil is invaluable for sufferers who need treatment, but cannot spare the time to physically relax. For instance, you can apply a little oil to your fingertips prior to taking a driving test and lose all of your tension while still being 100% alert ... wonderful! Not for nothing did the old-time herbalists say that Basil should be used to 'procure cheerful and merry hearts'. For elderly gentlemen suffering from 'heavy heads' and from blocked up sinuses, a pinch of powdered Basil taken as snuff will quickly and pleasantly remedy the situation. Basil also has another very good use in that 1 teaspoon added to a pan of boiling water and used to wash walls, floors, ceilings etc., is not only a good disinfectant but will also rid the home of 'malodorous humours' as they used to be called ... including the unwelcome odour of tom-cat which can be most distressing to say the least ... what a bountiful herb and how wonderful that it can be purchased for a few pence at the local store and kept fresh for months on the spice shelf.

Bayleaf

Since early Roman times Bay leaves have been used as a standard remedy for sore, chilled, damaged or aching limbs. In fact it was standard practice for Roman soldiers coming home from battle or long marches to sprinkle a handful of Bay leaves into their warm spring-water baths to ease their weary limbs and get them into a fit state, both physically and mentally to cope with the rigours of a quite different kind that were awaiting them after their long absences from home!

Be that as it may, the best use to which we may put our Bay leaves today is still to add a few crushed leaves to the bathwater to both relax our joints and stimulate our minds at the end of a busy, tiring or stressful day. However, I would recommend tying the crumpled leaves in a cloth or handkerchief before introducing to the bath to save getting covered in bits!

Bay leaves, when crumbled and thrown on the fire, also make a refreshing room purifier and disinfectant which is especially beneficial in rooms with stone floors or without damp-courses. A very efficacious Bay oil for massaging into joints which are afflicted with arthritis, rheumatism, fibrositis or similar aches and pains can be simply made by crushing about half a dozen Bay leaves or taking 1 flat teaspoon of powdered Bay and adding it to a small bottle of olive oil, shaking well, and keeping it in a warm place and using when needed. This oil will also lift the spirits if massaged into the soles of the feet!
In case the damage has already been done and a violent bout of indigestion is under way ... take heart ... Bay to the rescue!
Do make liberal use of Bay in cooking for inner ease as well, as its medicinal action on the digestive tract is well known. Bay

leaves have always been an important ingredient in bouquet garni for adding to soups, stuffings and roasting meats. Also, 1 leaf added to the water when poaching salmon will improve the flavour and impart a distinctive flavour, which will not only tempt the most jaded palate, but also ensure comfort at the end of the meal. This is a very good tip for flatulence sufferers! Simply put 1 or 2 well crushed Bayleaves or half a teaspoon of powdered Bay into a bowl of warm water and sit quietly bathing your feet in the bowl until the attack passes, topping up with water when needed to keep the feet really warm.

My father has not known many days in his life when he has not bathed his feet in this way, and he is still one of the sprightliest octogenarians I know, despite having only one lung. His statement on this is that "Your best friends are your feet and if you look after them, they'll look after you". How true!

Bay rum and Bay oil were once specifically used to cure sparse and falling hair and baldness, and they are still ingredients of many hair tonics available over the counter today ... if you wish to test the efficacy of this remedy, I suggest you try a little homemade Bay oil, rubbing with brisk circular movements into the offending area and leaving to penetrate for at least an hour before washing, then rinsing with rosemary or thyme mix.

Caraway

Caraway seeds are the seeds which we all remember our grandmothers putting into cakes and 'fairy buns' and feeding to us on Sunday afternoon visits 'if we behaved' ! Young people today do not relish these 'old-fashioned' cakes; would they, I wonder, change their tunes if they knew that the great Dioscorides in his time advised 'whey-faced girls' to take these seeds to keep their lovers from proving fickle!

Caraway was also an important ingredient to 'love potions', but I cannot make such extravagant claims today!

I can claim however, that Caraway is one of the nicest digestive aids to take, as it lends itself to many recipes and does not have to be taken 'as a medicine'. Baked apples, stuffed with mixed dried fruit to which a quarter of a teaspoon of Caraway seeds have been added, is one of the tastiest desserts after a rich or fatty meal, and one which ensures that no indigestion attacks follow the repast!

If you have young children constantly clamouring for some 'sweeties' and you know that they spend their pocket money on saccharine-based goodies which are not going to aid their digestion at all, make them some Caraway cornfits and stop worrying about the junk that they have when out of sight! To 1 stiffly beaten egg white, stir 1 heaped tablespoon of caster sugar and 1 oz of the seeds. Spread on a fine sieve and dry in a warm oven after baking ... kiddies love them!

As Caraway is such a good general tonic, it would be wise to take a little every day; that is why I feel so attuned to Caraway ... it can be taken in so many tasty ways.

A pinch of the seeds can be added to sandwiches, salads, cooked and raw vegetables, stocks, soups, stews, pies, jams, jellies, biscuits and cakes, enhancing their flavours and giving you the reputation of being a magnificent cook and hostess whose meals do not cause repercussions later in the day! All of the family would benefit from taking this tonic.

As another of Caraway's virtues is that it takes away the discomfort and the discoloration of bruising, it is wise to keep a bottle of Caraway oil in case of emergencies. Bruise 1 teaspoon of seeds and add to a small bottle of warmed sunflower oil. .. this is easily warmed by standing the bottle of oil in a bowl of hot water. .. stand the bottle in an easily accessible place, shaking daily, and massage into painful places as and when necessary.

This oil is also most beneficial to anyone suffering from bloating with flatulence or 'windy tummy' and brings swift relief if massaged into the stomach in a clockwise direction (i.e. from low right, up and over and down left side).

Earache can be eased, as can neuralgia and toothache, by pounding 1 teaspoon of seeds with a piece of stale bread or toast and adding a little boiling water to moisten, then putting the resultant mess into a clean piece of linen, cotton or muslin and applying to the aching place ... relief is almost immediate!

Cayenne pepper

Cayenne pepper is familiar to most of us in the kitchen as a useful additive to 'add a little bite' to savoury dishes.
In fact the word Cayenne comes from the Greek word 'to bite'!

This is a very useful condiment as, used in place of ordinary pepper, it can help to reduce dilated blood vessels and relieve chronic congestion ... this is especially helpful to heavy drinkers as they are often unaware of needing any medication until their condition is severe, so a little daily prevention will be better than a sudden need for a drastic cure.

As Cayenne is a powerful local stimulant, it really comes into its own when mixed into a cream, lard or oil base and applied as an ointment to areas which have become severely chilled, e.g. the muscles of fishermen who have been out all night enjoying the dubious pleasures of night-fishing, the knees of motor-cyclists after a long journey on a windy day, low back chills brought on by sitting in draughty school halls while watching the school play etc., etc.

To make, simply add 1 flat teaspoon of Cayenne to about 2 oz of vegetable lard (other bases can be used in a similar ratio if necessary) and heat very gently for about five minutes, stirring constantly ... pour into a small jar and allow to cool; you will then have an excellent embrocation. This ointment is very warming so should not be applied to very tender skin such as at the sides of the mouth, near the eyes, or particularly in any unmentionable places!

Cayenne is an excellent general stimulant and is very efficacious in building up resistance at the beginning of a cold, for this reason, it is often one of the ingredients of proprietary brands of cough medicine, digestifs and tonics.

It can also be obtained in powder or tablet form to help ease the discomfort of stomach and bowel cramps, which can at times be so very painful that not only are they disabling to the sufferer but can, quite understandably, give one the fear that they are suffering from very much more serious complaints and fear, causing as it does much more tension in the body, creates an ever increasing vicious circle of pain = fear = more pain.

Cayenne (or capsicum, chilli-pepper, Spanish or red pepper) serves another very useful purpose in that it stimulates the appetite and can be used in a variety of recipes, so does not have to be taken as a medicine, but can be enjoyed and even sought after by the sufferer, which is a real bonus.

Anorexia nervosa sufferers have been known to enjoy a dish of artistically prepared red-yellow-green capsicums or a salad containing them and, containing as they do large quantities of many of the vitamins so necessary to good health and recovery from illness without any of the dreaded fattening properties, they should form a regular place in every anorexic's diet and would hasten their recovery.

I cannot stress too strongly how good Cayenne is in this respect and would advise anyone who has a sufferer from loss of appetite in their family to use Cayenne pepper regularly.

Loss of taste can be a very difficult problem to deal with. One way in which we can help ourselves to restore it is to make the Dr's Taste Reviver, which is very simply a good pinch of Cayenne pepper added to a cup of hot water with a little sea salt and a knob of butter added. This makes a very tasty drink to take in all wintry conditions and stimulates the taste buds; anyone who has lost their capacity for enjoying their food will soon find that it returns if they keep taking the tonic. For anyone suffering from a weak digestion who loves pickles and chutneys but regrets indulging in them for hours afterwards, Cayenne could be the answer to your dilemma. Here is a chutney which will help and not hinder digestion:

Mince together 1 peeled cucumber, 1 Spanish onion, 1 head of garlic (anyone who does not like garlic can substitute a shallot), add 1 tablespoon of lemon or lime juice and a quarter of a teaspoon of Cayenne; blend together well, bottle and use when the temptation to have chutney or pickle is too strong to resist! Chilblain sufferers will also have cause to bless Cayenne, for an application to increase the poor circulation which caused them and is very simply made by adding 1 teaspoon of Cayenne to half a cup of boiling water, cooling and keeping in the refrigerator and applying daily after bathing.

One of the most widespread disorders in the world is also one of the most difficult to treat due to its being caused by so many different catalysts. However, I can state from personal experience that the above mixture, applied hot, brings blessed relief from that scourge of mankind ... RHEUMATISM ... what a godsend!

Celery

Celery is one of the best known natural healers for those dreadfully debilitating, ageing and painful complaints ...

rheumatism and rheumatoid arthritis. It restores lost tissue, nerve and muscle tone, expels surplus fluids from between the tissues which can both cause and result from nervous tension. It is both a relaxant and a stimulant as and when needed, and is a good guard against insomnia ... what a wonderful medicine.

Although, strictly speaking, Celery and its virtues should be discussed in volume four 'The Vegetable Rack', it is available in dried, seed and salt form, therefore, no respectable spice shelf should be without at least one of these items:
Celery is one of the best known natural healers for those dreadfully debilitating, ageing and painful complaints ... rheumatism and rheumatoid arthritis. It restores lost tissue, nerve and muscle tone, expels surplus fluids from between the tissues which can both cause and result from nervous tension. It is both a relaxant and a stimulant as and when needed, and is a good guard against insomnia ... what a wonderful medicine.

Celery salt is plentiful, relatively inexpensive and also very pleasant tasting; therefore it is simple to help yourself with Celery by substituting it for ordinary salt both in cooking and on the meal table. How marvellous to be able to ease aches and pains by simply changing our condiments!
Celery soup can be made instantly and very cheaply by adding a good pinch of Celery salt to a cup of hot water; this makes a

great stimulant throughout the day, especially when joints are chilled, yet promotes soothing sleep when taken at night. Celery seeds are also readily available and can be added to soups, stews, dumplings etc. in winter. .. salads in summer. .. or just chewed as and when required to bring relief. Celery tea bags can also be used for all of the above.

Chervil & Chives

There are of course many recipes that call for one of these herb-spices and many cooks use them regularly without realising that they too have their medicinal uses.

Chervil's effect is toning and as a blood purifier, what could be simpler than to add a little of the chopped herb or seeds to a salad, to vegetables as a garnish or to butter or sauces.
In Europe, chopped Chervil is chopped into bread dough where its distinctive aroma and taste make the 'Provence loaf' a much sought-after delicacy ... As Chervil is also reputed to stimulate the brain, I feel that that is reason enough to often indulge in a ploughman's lunch consisting of home-made Chervil bread (I sometimes cheat here and buy a commercially prepared bread-mix and add a teaspoonful of chopped seeds ... the results are perfect every time!) some small onions or garlic cloves and a

cup of cottage cheese liberally laced with Chives. If my nerves are frayed or I am feeling a little depressed, a cup of Chervil tea (made by soaking a pinch of dried leaves or crushed seeds in a cup of boiling water) soon has me 'on top of things' and has the added advantage of moderately warming the stomach, thus aiding digestion and promoting a feeling of 'well-being'. Chives really need no introduction as we all use them at some time or other as an addition to salads, chopped into omelettes, cheeses, soups, sauces and savoury dishes, sprinkled into sandwiches or yogurts, etc ... but ... don't forget Chives' main virtue, if you need garlic but find it too strong ... change to Chives.

Cinnamon

Cinnamon has long had the reputation of strengthening the 'enfeebled stomach', hence its addition in the making of rich cakes, pastries and puddings. In the Far
East it is very often added to rich meat dishes, as it is renowned there for combating the effects of too much grease in the digestive tract.

I find that people who say 'l love lamb and mutton but they don't like me' can take them with impunity if half of a teaspoon of Cinnamon is added during cooking ... the flavour is delicious. If this has been forgotten, the distension and discomfort that follows can speedily be dispelled by adding a good pinch of Cinnamon to a teacup of hot water and sipping slowly ... you can also add the same amount or a Cinnamon stick to a pot of tea, then add milk and sweetener and drink any time to strengthen the digestive tract, to calm and soothe and to generally promote a feeling of well-being.

Because of its relaxant properties, the above tea, taken before a journey, acts very effectively against travel sickness and acts quickly to relieve nauseous and bilious headaches. All of us at some time in our lives either have experienced, or are going to experience, the 'sickness at food' which is really the natural defence system of the body letting us know that our stomachs need a rest ... to nourish the body while letting it rest, yet at the same time satisfying our minds that we are doing all that we can to help ourselves, is very easy with the help of this wonderworking tea in place of a few meals.

Childbirth is sometimes followed by a host of attendant discomforts, not least being an inordinately long period of bleeding after the birth sometimes accompanied by discomfort and occasionally by mild local infections which can create great distress if not cleared up quickly.

A Cinnamon wash with its antiseptic properties, can be a quick and effective way of alleviating these problems:

To half a pint of warm water add half a teaspoon of Cinnamon ... using cotton-wool balls dipped in the mixture, wash around the vagina then taking a tampon, quickly immerse in the mixture and insert while still warm. This should be done every time that the tampon needs changing until the trouble has cleared up. If tampons are not used, add Cinnamon to the bath water as well as bathing affected parts every time sanitary pads are changed.

Another attendant discomfort which follows not only childbirth but also operations, enforced bed rest and any other period of inactivity which can interfere with our digestion, is WIND ... or to put it more politely ... spontaneous flatulence!

This must surely be one of the most embarrassing, uncomfortable and infuriating complaints on this planet. .. it is certainly the one which provokes the least amount of sympathy and the most ridiculous jokes and cretinous remarks ... but help is at hand! Simply add quarter of a teaspoon of Cinnamon to quarter of a teacupful of hot water and take BEFORE meals to prevent occurrences and, in stubborn cases, take between meals to expel wind and bloating from the system in a very short time.

Babies, young children, and elderly and infirm people often have a lot of trouble accepting full meals at times when their digestive systems are undergoing change. This can be quickly eliminated by the addition of a powdering of Cinnamon on the top of a cup of warm milk which has been sweetened with honey given in place of one meal a day for a few days ... I found that this drink, taken at bedtime, promoted a deep sleep and a healthy appetite the next day with no repercussions!

In times of dire emergency when babies and young children are suddenly afflicted with violent diarrhoea in the middle of the night, or when grand ad is taken with a fit of vomiting because of indulging himself with 'the lads' at the local, Cinnamon really proves its worth ... in fact, it is priceless!

Mix together quarter of a teaspoon of Cinnamon and 1 tablespoon of corn flour in 3-4 tablespoons of milk, stir well and drink quickly to coat and soothe the stomach ... this is an invaluable and infallible remedy ... if you do not use either Cinnamon or corn flour for any other purpose than this, I feel that they still earn their places on your spice shelf on this merit alone.

Highly regarded from ancient times, it is even referred to in the Bible as one of the ingredients of the Holy Anointing Oil (Ex.30.23) and as an aphrodisiac (Prov.7.17) it was also one of the herbs for which Crusades were mounted in order to import them in the Middle Ages. Men have fought and died for the right to own Cinnamon yet, now it is so readily available, it is sadly neglected in our medicine chests ... we must remedy this!

Cloves

Cloves are a germicide, antiseptic and local anaesthetic and are also purported to be a stimulant of the parts that other remedies cannot reach, so it really does seem wasteful of their properties if all we do with them is to flavour apple pies!

The main use to which I put Cloves when my children were small was to banish the pain caused by cutting their teeth, and, as at one time I had four children with the eldest being only four years old, it is easy to imagine the amount of teething that went on in our house ... it was non-stop ... However, we coped with the minimum of pain to babies and strain to parents thanks to the judicious use of Cloves.

I would most strongly advise anyone with small babies to get themselves a bottle of Clove oil the next time they visit the chemist, which simply has to be applied as and when needed. But in cases of emergency, our Cloves on the spice shelf will serve every bit as well, not only for babies teething, but also for anyone who is suffering from the torments of toothache. A seed of whole Clove can be placed in the cavity of an aching tooth to warm and relieve the pain quickly, a cotton-wool bud moistened and dipped into powdered Cloves then applied to the affected part and bitten down on will work the same way (be careful not to touch the lips with this as it is HOT!). A pinch of powdered Cloves mixed with a teaspoon of honey can be rubbed into sore and inflamed gums to cool and soothe. This acts as a local anaesthetic which acts quickly and surely.

There are a lot of complaints which can be greatly alleviated by the application of a warming ointment which will soothe the pain brought on by muscle spasms, not the least of these being the simple cramp which strikes with no warning, doubles us up with pain, and for which the recommended proprietary brand of tablets advise 'take half an hour before the cramps occur'. I never have been able to figure out the logic of that instruction! A champion and deeply penetrating ointment can be easily and inexpensively made as follows:

To 1 lb (or 500 kg) of vegetable lard add 1 oz (or 25 gms) of dried powdered Cloves. Put in covered ovenproof dish (or similar ovenproof) container and cook on a low heat for about 1 hour (I usually pop this on the bottom shelf of the oven at the same time as I cook my slow-roast, this way it utilises some oven space and time). Take out VERY CAREFULLY, stir thoroughly and allow to cool for about an hour before straining through a cloth into screw-top jars. Do not put the lids on until this is absolutely cold and set, then keep in the refrigerator until needed.

This ointment can be used to warm and soothe pains caused by chilled or cramped muscles, hypothermia, frostbite, lumbago, influenza, neuralgia, pleurisy, rheumatism, sciatica and all related aches and pains which need an external application of heat ... but beware ... NEVER APPLY TO BROKEN SKIN as this is such a HOT mixture! Also, AL WAYS wash your hands immediately after applying, as the thoughtless touch of this cream to intimate areas and tender skin can be very uncomfortable!

Coriander & Cumin

Coriander is another aromatic spice-herb which we owe to the Romans, as they recognised its soothing properties and its ability to disguise the taste of foods which were perhaps not so fresh as they should be, or medicines which were bitter. Although we would not dream of putting it to the former use today, it can still provide very useful as an addition to medicines which would be unpalatable without it, e.g. senna, gentian etc.

One of my many aunts used to make 'sweeties' for us as children by mixing an ounce of Coriander seeds into a little pot with icing sugar and a little water, then allowing us to separate the stickilycovered seeds and put them in a warm place to dry. As we very often ate most of the 'comfits' in the process, I feel sure that, unbeknown to us, we were in need of a tonic and this was her way of ensuring that we took one ... how much nicer that was than taking a spoonful of nasty medicine, and how effective. I have found that the crushed seeds made into a poultice with a little bread and hot water can be a very soothing dressing for erysipelas, any itching or burning skin and inflamed arthritis.

Cumin has a very bitter flavour which would be enhanced by the addition of a little Coriander (although my grandfather's way of spreading a little olive-oil on bread, which he then sprinkled with powdered Cumin and munched with obvious relish between glasses of home-made 'porter', seems the very best way that one could possibly take this medicine!). Used in curries and sauces, if you need caraway or fennel and do not have any ... use Cumin.

Dill

Dill is one of the earliest medicinal herbs known in Europe; a very similar herb in its actions to anise, It is especially good for easing hiccoughs in young children so has been used for centuries as the main ingredient in soothing syrups and gripe-waters.

The essential oil which Dill yields and which can be obtained from any good health food store, contains hydrocarbons and oxygenated oil and forms a champion remedy for dispelling wind which has become trapped in the bowels and which, as any sufferer knows, creates a terribly painful situation and one which provokes no sympathy from non-sufferers!
Unlike wind in the digestive tract which one often recognises for what it is, in the bowel the pain can radiate to such an extent that one can be certain that something very serious is amiss, creating a pain = fear = tension = increased pain syndrome which can lead to very severe problems both for the sufferer and those around them. If you have anyone in the family home who suffers from this complaint (and I do mean SUFFERS), make sure that you have some Dill seeds on your spice shelf. To make a quick and effective remedy, simply crush 1 flat teaspoon of Dill seeds, add boiling water and stir well; when at a suitable temperature for drinking, add honey to taste and sip slowly.. - as with all long-standing complaints, this remedy will need to be taken quite regularly to begin with, but once the symptoms ease off, it will not need to be taken so often and, as with all remedies, only take until symptoms stop.

Fennel

As a child I often picked the feathery fronds of Fennel on the Cornish cliffs near the sea and took them home to put in a vase in my bedroom where I was told that they would stop me from having bad dreams, but in reality, their aroma eased my breathing and disinfected my room bringing peaceful sleep!

I was also told by my great-aunt Boadicea that the Fennel plant was 'our family plant' having been brought into Europe by the great Charlemagne from whom our family are said to have descended... Fennel was apparently one of the first crops for which farmers were given a subsidy for growing, as it was esteemed by Charlemagne as an excellent food, medicine and wine plant, and it was cultivated on all the Imperial farms.
Be that as it may, I have found over the years that Fennel is absolutely indispensible in our home ... it is a wonderful healer for disease of what I term the 'yellow' areas of the body ... stomach, spleen, pancreas, gall-bladder, liver, kidneys etc., in fact all the organs which can be found in an area covered by a handspan around the body above the navel.
It has been my contention for some time that almost all of the diseases known to man have their organic roots in this area, 'in

our middles' as a little friend once put it ... out of the mouths of babes indeed ... if we get our 'middles' right then everything else will soon be in tip-top form also, and with a sense of responsibility and care for ourselves and with Fennel freely available, we can start repairing right away.

Fennel is the most infallible treatment for obesity in the world today, yet is the most little used remedy on the market for this complaint ... probably due to its cheapness! Sometimes I wish that I could take the most 'hopeless' cases and keep them under my care for a few months: feeding them on unadulterated food and giving them Fennel in copious quantities would, I am sure, have a remarkable effect.

Anyone suffering from the effects of a sluggish metabolism should immediately replace the drinking of tea and coffee with Fennel; also, take Fennel as a vegetable and chew the seeds ... the effect on the body will be noticeable almost immediately! The seeds are very tasty and have the added bonus of cleansing the breath while acting as a diuretic ... the plants were often grown by the doorway of Quaker meeting houses to enable early 'Friends' to chew them in their meetings and early settlers in America called them 'Meeting seeds'.

Very often the cause of obesity can be what used to be called 'tired blood' ... this is no longer a fashionable or acceptable description for what is still a very real and nasty complaint, yet if our bloodstream has to carry a lot of chemical residues and our circulation becomes impaired as a result, allowing water to lodge between body tissues and in our veins, tired blood can very aptly describe the condition ... However, as another of Fennel's virtues is its blood cleansing property, it is easy to understand my enthusiasm for the use of this wonderful herb. No spice shelf should be without these tasty and useful seeds. Fennel tea is simply and quickly made by pouring half a pint of boiling water over 1 teaspoon of bruised seeds and stirring vigorously, then allowing to settle for a few minutes until it is at drinking temperature, seasoning or sweetening to taste and drinking at any times of the day or night as required. This tea can be taken to ease any of the following:

Infant's colic, flatulence, stones in gall-bladder or kidneys, pancreatitis, nausea, jaundice, cramp, gout and arthritis.

To make a very effective gripe-water for infants, simply add 1 teaspoon of honey and a good pinch of bicarbonate of soda to the above tea, stirring vigorously for one whole minute, then straining and bottling. This can be refrigerated when cold and administered in teaspoonful doses as and when required. Alternatively, crush 1 heaped teaspoon of Fennel seeds and add to a jar of clear honey,

Stir well and keep the jar in a very warm place and add 1 teaspoon of Fennel honey to a cup of hot water when required ... this is a good standby to keep in the store cupboard for emergencies, as it also makes a quick flavouring for cakes, biscuits, salad-dressings etc.

Fennel has yet another very great virtue that is invaluable: it has the ability to restore failing vision ... surely this is a most wonderful and priceless product . . . wonderful indeed, yet costing only pence and readily available at the supermarket and even in

Some small country stores, it constantly amazes me how little it is used or appreciated. Simply strain plain Fennel tea to make a most efficacious eyewash and use every night.

Garlic

Garlic is strictly speaking a vegetable and as such, its many virtues will be fully covered in the volume entitled 'The Vegetable Rack'. However, as powdered and granulated Garlic can be kept on the spice shelf, I will say a few words in its favour now (if I can keep my enthusiasm for it in check!)

First and foremost, I cannot stress too strongly that there is no other single herb which does such a sterling job as an antiseptic and purifier of the bloodstream ... I do not feel that I am exaggerating when I state that it is thanks mainly to Garlic that I am alive and well today.

Once, while recovering from a fall which created a situation where I was unable to take my daily dose of Garlic for eighteen months, I became so stiff in my joints, obese, and infection prone that I vowed never again to let a day go by without taking a capsule of Garlic on retiring to keep myself in top form.

As The Good Book states. . . 'The life of all things is in the blood' ... and if the blood is full of impurities which it has to carry around our bodies for 24 hours of each day, it stands to reason that it will be unable to function at 100% of its capacity ... would you be able to do your daily work efficiently if you were carrying a sack of potatoes or a double armful of books? .. This is, in effect, what we ask our bodies to do! Now, thanks to Garlic, you will no longer have to do this.

All of us are familiar with the one drawback which prevents Garlic from taking its rightful place as the most used herb/vegetable in our larders ... the odour! However, chewing a juicy apple or a sprig of parsley after eating Garlic will make sure that the breath is sweet and clean again, *so,* bearing that in mind, we really should make the effort to incorporate more Garlic into our day to- day recipes.

If you are not used to cooking with Garlic, try first of all introducing just a little to the cooking-pot when making soups or stews. Alternatively, have some Garlic salt on the table and sprinkle it on steak, sausages or salads ... you will be surprised at the flavour-enhancing properties of this herb. A little every day will gradually clear the bloodstream and start to build up the strength of anyone at any age who has been suffering from the effects of toxins in the bloodstream. . . tiredness and lassitude, constipation, biliousness, headaches, lank or splitting hair, itching, spotty or scaly skin, warts, corns and verrucae, coughs and colds which recur regularly, cystitis, irregular periods, morbid fears or depression, gouty arthritis, rheumatism and hard swollen joints to name but a few. What an amazing remedy this is to bring effective relief from so many ailments in such a pleasant and simple way ... no doubt this is why so many of the old herbal simples are so called ... because the remedies are just that ... yet I do not know of many other remedies that are so all-embracing and complete in their treatment as my very good friend Garlic.

One of the many ways in which Garlic proved such a good friend to me when my children were little and spending almost as much time 'in the wars' as they did playing, was as an antiseptic and ever-ready 'cure-all' to apply to their everyday injuries, and, having as I did, four youngsters all in the same age range, these occurred with inevitable regularity!

Anyone having small children would be well advised to give them their own personal 'Garlic-Rescue' to carry around with them ... mine each had a small plastic salt or pepper pot full to carry in their pockets with instructions to use it absolutely any

time that they felt the need of it ... and used it certainly was! Bites, stings, scratches, grazes, burns, scalds, all were quite liberally sprinkled with this 'magic mixture', then play continued without the nuisance of having to go home and have their 'wounds' attended in the middle of their adventures ...
Those little pots of powdered Garlic and a few plasters gave me peace of mind no matter where my children were playing and allowed them quite a lot more freedom to roam than they would have had without them.

In some of the busiest hospitals in China and Japan, where limb and organ transplants are performed daily on a grand scale as a matter of routine, very often the only antiseptic applied after stitching is ... Garlic! If it can be relied on for such truly important matters, surely we should be ashamed of ourselves if we do not take advantage of its wonderful properties and keep it ever handy on our spice shelf.

Ginger

Cultivated as it is in the West Indies, Africa and Jamaica, it is hardly surprising that Ginger is so wonderfully hot, spicy and delicious ... yet its flavour is only one facet of its value; it is also a valuable remedy to keep on our increasingly useful spice shelf.

While making their voyages of discovery in the East Indies, the Spaniards realised what a valuable food remedy Ginger had been to the natives for centuries, so they transplanted some and took it to Spain for cultivation, where it flourished so vigorously that, by 1547, they had exported over 22,000 cwt into Europe! In the Middle Ages when a woman was queen in the home, and the kitchen, or rather the dishes which issued from it, reflected her prowess as such, happy indeed was the woman who had a stock of such a fine spice and many the delicious meal, cordial or simple proudly presented to guests as 'containing 'Asian-root".

Since that time, Ginger has been increasingly and regularly used to delight the palate, soothe the stomach and digestive tract, ease the throat and chest, cleanse the system of parasites and infections, regulate menses, warm and relax when chilled and, of course, enhance the flavour of a variety of beverages, not least being the 'water of life' of the Celts!

Being available in so many forms, Ginger can be kept in every home without much fear of it being 'left on the shelf' for very long ... fresh, crystallised, candied or bottled root, dried whole or powdered root are readily available in most stores.

Ginger is much in evidence in my home in a variety of forms, as I find it invaluable for the prevention of so many 'niggling' ailments which can affect anyone of any age whose system is not kept clear and whose 'humours' are not kept free-flowing! Being a very busy person with very little time to spare, the versatility of Ginger pleases me greatly ... As a preventive measure of tummy upsets which so often occur with the change of the seasons, it is second to none for ease of use ... I simply keep some crystallised and candied Ginger freely available on the coffee table where anyone who has a mind to, can 'take their medicine' in passing without even realising that they have done so. The men in my family seem to take this more than anyone else and, as the male sex generally are the hardest to advise or treat regarding their eating habits and the results of not taking care of them, this is quite a boon to me!

Men are also the ones who are most likely to go out in the biting wind without a coat or stay out overnight fishing when it is pouring with rain etc., etc. The very best way to ensure that such foolhardiness does not result in sniffly colds, thick heads or sore throats, sinus problems, swollen joints or any of the numerous complaints from which we are led to believe that the sufferer will surely die, is to greet them on their return with a greatly appreciated and very efficacious glass of green Ginger wine or cordial.

.. either hot, cold, straight or mixed ... the medicinal effect is just as strong and the psychological effect can sometimes be even stronger, as the man who is glad to be home can resist ailments easier than a 'nagged' one!

Anyone who has small children or aged relatives to cope with would be well advised to keep dried Ginger always in the house, as it is an invaluable remedy for diarrhoea, flatulence and colic which so often affect people in the extreme age ranges. One of the beauties of this remedy is that it is cheap, readily available, and tasty to take ... I almost always have Ginger cake in my tin, as a slice of this should be quite sufficient to clear up the offending complaint (although most sufferers will insist that they need another dose!).

Another tasty way to obtain speedy relief from any of the above symptoms is to add half a teaspoon to a pot of tea and slowly sip and savour a cup which has been sweetened with honey to taste.

Ginger tea, when used as a gargle, can be of great comfort to anyone suffering from a sore throat, loss of voice or toothache, and also brings relief from toothache and neuralgia if applied unsweetened as a poultice or fomentation; an easy way to apply this is to soak a flannel or piece of cotton/linen in the tea, then wring out and apply to the painful place, covering with a hot water- bottle or hot-pack which can be inexpensively obtained at most large stores (they are usually intended to keep frozen goods cold or picnic meals hot).

Rheumatism, cramp, 'frozen' and stiff joints will all respond very well to these fomentations.

Painful or irregular periods cause a lot of problems, yet these too can be speedily eased with this little wonder-worker. .. try taping a slice of root Ginger over the umbilicus (a plaster patch is ideal for this) ... Ginger quickly brings relief. Aahhh!

MACE

Mace is actually the outer husk of the Myristica Officinalis, of which the inner seed is known to us as nutmeg and, as a general rule, their actions are similar ... Mace outside, nutmeg inside.

Although Mace is a versatile and tasty spice which lends itself to the preparation of so many recipes, both sweet and savoury, the use to which I put it to more times than any other is to bring speedy relief to sufferers of gout, rheumatism and arthritis.
It is simplicity itself to make an ointment, which will keep for up to a few months if refrigerated, by melting together:
1 teaspoon of powdered Mace with 2-3 oz (or 50-75 gm) of vegetable lard, heating on lowest possible heat for approximately half an hour, then stirring well and bottling when cool.

This ointment should be well massaged into the affected joints or muscles after bathing or washing in very warm water, and preferably before retiring, as it will then penetrate deeply and have all night to perform its healing action and be much more efficacious.

This works particularly well in cases of gouty-arthritis which do not respond well to any other treatment ...

This is the case with so many of these spice remedies as they are often not tried until all else has failed ... what a shame it seems to me that we all have the makings of vibrant good health in our larders and so many times do not make enough use of them.

However, that will now be remedied as you use this little book to help you utilise your 'Marvellous Mace'!

If there is no time to make the ointment and the sufferer feels that they just cannot cope with the pain any longer, put 1 teaspoon of dried powdered Mace into a pot and pour on 1 pint (or half a litre) of boiling water, stir. Use a little poured onto a cloth, sponge or flannel and apply to the affected part as a soothing fomentation.

This can also be used to very quickly ease cramp and colicy pains in the stomach which often accompany fevers.

This mixture can be poured into a bowl of hot water and the feet bathed in it to bring lasting ease to sufferers of gout or bunions, it is especially efficacious if at the same time the sufferer uses a cup of the mixture to drink as a tea with a little honey to sweeten if required ... the relief is bliss.

As Mace is also very good for regulating the circulation and especially for calming when the heart is racing during fevers and times of digestive upheavels, it can prove invaluable to mothers of young children (as I found out when my four all seemed to share their ailments with each other, giving me quadruple problems to deal with).

To ease fevers, calm upset stomachs and warm the system gently, simply mix quarter of a teaspoon of powdered Mace with 1 teaspoon of honey and add to a cup of warm milk. .. this is especially good when taken at bedtime and brings restful healing sleep. Although Mace is so good for all these problems, for me at least, its main virtue must be as an infallible remedy for cramps;

Mace bags made like lavender bags and worn in a sock while sleeping, soon make cramp a thing of the past ... Magic Mace!

Marjoram

Marjoram must surely have been one of the earliest herbs used, as seeds of it have been found in the interglacial deposits near Clacton in the UK dating from approximately 160,000 years ago. The ancient Greeks cultivated Marjoram on their hillsides, taking hives there in the summer so that their honey would carry not only the medicinal properties of Marjoram, but it's delicious flavour which was much sought after.

Marjoram's botanical name, Origanum, means in fact 'mountains of beauty or joy' and both Greek and Roman lovers wore betrothal crowns of Marjoram ... Marjoram was also planted on the graves of loved ones and if the plants flourished, it proved that the dead were happy in the next world and everyone rejoiced.

Many a time, I rejoiced as a child when entering the dwelling of Granny Orchard; to see and smell the fragrant bunches of herbs which hung from the ceiling, and to be treated to a cup of sweet smelling and even sweeter tasting tea when feeling all hot, bothered and grumpy soon made the world seem right again!

I realise now that the 'measles spot tea' and 'fever foot wash' which made me feel so much better, also the ingredient in the little 'bath bags' which were made by Granny Orchard reaching up into her fragrant ceiling, picking a handful of the herbs there and tying them into a 'hanky' while telling me that these were soothing for 'tired bones, old bones, nerve bones and lazy bones', must have been the herb of joy and beauty, Marjoram. These bath bags are very efficacious in soothing frayed nerves. Marjoram is not often used in herbalism today, but more as a culinary herb, which to my mind is a great pity as it is very useful especially to the mothers of small children.

One of its many uses is as a stimulant which induces a gentle perspiration and brings out the eruptions at the commencement of measles ... this is a blessing indeed as until the spots show themselves no one can be absolutely sure of the cause of the high fever and irritability which are apparent in the child at the onset of this illness.

It is also useful for easing all dyspepsic complaints including gastric headaches, colic, liver upsets and dropsical conditions and also a sovereign remedy for easing period pains, releasing a stopped menstrual flow and lifting the depression of PMT.

Another of Marjoram's many uses is that of soother to lungs which have been overworked by the laboured breathing of asthma, bronchitis, catarrh and emphysema.

To bring ease to the sufferer of any of the above complaints, a pinch of dried Marjoram in a cup of boiling water or 1 teaspoon of dried leaves or powder added to a pot, makes a soothing and tasty drink which is very readily assimilated by the body and which quickly brings relief.

This tea, if applied externally as a cold poultice, is excellent for taking down swellings and easing the painful swollen joints that are so excruciating for arthritis and rheumatism sufferers; also, strains, sprains, torn ligaments and bruising respond well to being dressed with bandages soaked in this poultice.

Mint

Of all the herbs available for our use today, Mint must surely be the most unappreciated ... introduced into Britain by the Romans as a medicine herb, if grown in the garden it usually does not need much encouragement to run wild and then we rush to dig it up, cut it down, burn it, bury it or otherwise dispose of it as completely as possible ... Then we often bemoan the fact that our back aches from gardening and we do not have a remedy at hand ... what about the marvellous properties of Mint!

Since the earliest records left by man, Mint in all forms has been used as a medicine for all manner of complaints, and it was listed in the ninth century as being available as a 'phyficke' in at least seven different forms as the apothecary women used fresh Mint, dry herbs, Mint water, Mint syrup, Mint conserve, Mint spirit and
Mint oil in simple or chemical form! Mint has been found wild in almost every country to which civilisation has extended, which to my mind, proves how well nature provides for us no matter where we are on this planet.

As Mint is a good remedy for enough ailments to merit a book to itself, I shall briefly list these ailments then list a few ways in which you may like to take it, but do experiment with Mint, as it is so readily available even if only on your spice shelf ... ready?

Abdominal complaints, arthritis, acne, cramps, coughs, colds, colic, fevers, headaches, heartburn, inflammation, insomnia, itching, menstrual problems, nausea, nervousness, PMT, rheumatism, stress and tension can all be relieved with Mint! Make sure that you are never without Mint on YOUR spice shelf!

Mint is one of the finest oxygenators of the bloodstream known to mankind and as such it is invaluable in assisting the healing of all circulatory disorders such as chaps, chilblains, erysipelas, haemorrhoids, varicose veins and wandering pains as well as the preceding list, and, for the ease of all such complaints an application of Mint ointment is recommended.

To make this inexpensive, sweet smelling and very useful cream or ointment simply take 1 cup of finely chopped fresh Mint, put into a glass or enamel baking dish (I often use my heat resistant jug for this with a small plate on the top as a loose lid), cover with half a pound or 250 gm of pure vegetable lard or solidified sunflower oil, cover and cook slowly on the bottom of the oven for 1 hour at 150-180 degrees ... It is most important not to have the oven heat too high, or the finished ointment will smell 'fatty', also to allow the steam to escape while cooking as this helps the keeping properties of the finished ointment. (Small amounts of this can be made very quickly during extreme emergencies by covering 1 teaspoon of dried Mint with 2 oz (or 50 gm) of vegetable lard and cooking in the microwave on medium power for 10 minutes ... this does not keep for any length of time but can be extremely useful as first-aid in a hurry). After removing from the heat and allowing to cool slightly, if the mixture is strained through a fine cloth into screw-topped jars and kept in the refrigerator, it can serve a double purpose, as it is not only an excellent ointment to ease many pains, but also an unusual condiment for use with many savoury dishes.

Speaking of condiments, most of us have a jar of commercially prepared Mint sauce base on our spice shelves, yet only use this as an accompaniment to roast lamb ... what a waste!

As this has a vinegar base, it can be a great help in adjusting the acid mantle of our skin, which, if it becomes too alkali, presents us with a variety of symptoms, the most troublesome being dry, flaky or itchy skin, dandruff, etc. it also discourages mites and head-lice which are so prevalent with young children (and certainly smells more pleasant than most commercial preparations in use for this purpose!).

Simply add 1 cup of boiling hot vinegar to either 1 heaped teaspoon of either commercially prepared Mint sauce base or 1 teaspoon of dried Mint, stir well and allow to cool, stirring regularly ... strain, bottle and keep tightly sealed for use as a scalp rub and rinse mixture for the above complaints.

Usually 1 tablespoon of this Mint vinegar rubbed well into the scalp about an hour before washing the hair will clear the scalp of all troubles, while the same amount added to 2 litres of warm water and used as the final rinse will discourage further 'unwanted visitors' leaving the hair beautifully soft and shining and better able to resist atmospheric pollution. An egg cupful of this mixture added to the bathwater instead of any commercial preparation not only very speedily clears up skin complaints but also has the benefit of being wonderfully invigorating as well, so is great for restoring energy at the end of a busy day ... a spoonful of Mint goes a long, long way!

Mint vinegar, when taken in hot water and sweetened with honey to taste makes a very tasty and effective medicinal drink to help ease all upsets which have their origin in the digestive tract ... even irritable bowel syndrome and diverticulitis respond well to this remedy which is commonly known as a toddy.

Another very common problem which affects the British race more than any other seems to be 'chesty and phlegmy coughs' ... these seem to affect everyone, regardless of age or circumstance, and hang around for a very long time unless 'nipped in the bud' ... Mint toddy, taken as above and drunk as hot as possible, will encourage the body to throw out its toxins quickly and promote a healthy perspiration to rid the body of its waste. This toddy is best taken at bedtime giving, it plenty of time to work while the body rests and repairs itself.

Infants respond particularly well to this Mint toddy when they are teething and it can be given warm as a soothing drink to cool fevers, or frozen into ice-cubes and rubbed on swollen gums when it eases the pain very quickly, bringing relief to baby and mother at the same time!

Sufferers from halitosis, sore gums and throats, abscesses in the mouth and similar complaints will be very pleased to hear that 1 tablespoonful of Mint vinegar added to 1 cup of cold water makes an excellent mouthwash and gargle which does not just mask the problem, as do so many commercial preparations, but gets to the root of the problem and by oxygenating the bloodstream, purifies and eliminates the cause ... marvellous!

Of course the most simple way to take Mint as a general tonic is to drink Mint-tea which is refreshing, soothing and very tasty.

Although this can be bought in loose or tea-bag form, if we have dried Mint on the spice shelf, all we need to do is to add a pinch of this to a cup of hot water or 1 teaspoonful to a pot and we have a quick 'pick-me-up' literally at our fingertips! This Mint tea strengthens the nerves and sinews, oxygenates the blood, eases flatulence, giddiness, hiccoughs, allays nausea and vomiting, clears the sinuses and, most important to my mind, helps to dispell those awful wandering pains, headaches and tensions associated with PMT, the menopause or STRESS. What a boon it is, for what could be more simple than to have a cuppa ... yet there are not many remedies that are so effective! This same tea, when used in an eye-bath is a very good cure for sties, conjunctivitis, etc.; also it is a very effective eye-wash for removing 'foreign bodies' (as a child I never could understand how anyone could get a foreign body in their eye and always looked in vain to see them brought out!)

Adding half an ounce of dried Mint to the tea caddy if one uses loose tea is an easy way of ensuring that all the family will benefit from the properties of this wonderful herb It is also nice to be able to offer friends who visit such a refreshing drink. All of the internal complaints listed can be helped by simply drinking Mint tea. However, many external inflammations also can be helped by soaking a cloth, flannel or bandage in Mint tea, wringing out, applying as hot as possible to the affected part, and sitting quietly for a little while ... you doubt? .. try it! Children often have tummy-upsets due to eating all sorts of 'junk food' while they are out playing or at school or with friends and we would be attempting the impossible by telling them only to eat wholesomely, therefore I have found a couple of ways in which I can give them preventive medicine

pleasantly. Mint cookies are very quickly made by mixing 3 oz (or 75 gm) flour, 3 oz (or 75 gm) porridge oats, 3 oz (or 75 gm) cane sugar and 4 oz (or 100 gm) pure vegetable lard with one small jar or 2 tablespoons of
Mint jelly and a little water until the mixture is bound into a pastry consistency. Rolled out, cut into shapes, moistened and sprinkled with sugar, these cookies can be baked on gas mark 5 or electric 200°C for 15 minutes, or in the microwave on high for 5 minutes ... Mmmmmm ... delicious.

Dried Mint can be easily powdered in a coffee grinder, then, if added to equal amounts of powdered cinnamon, cloves, fennel, nutmeg or mace and rosemary, can make a tasty alternative to the
Mint jelly in cookies. Also it can be used in muffins, buns and cakes; just add 1 heaped teaspoonful of the mixture to the cookie mixture or your usual recipe.

If this dried Mint/herb mixture is stored in a coffee jar until required, it can be used as any other instant drink powder in hot milk or water sweetened to taste. This makes a delicious and very effective intestinal warmer if anyone has stayed out in the wet or cold too long, or sat on damp grass or cold stone floors (I have also found this extremely effective for the men in my family who have sat on a riverbank in the freezing rain all day drowning worms and calling it 'great sport').

The Mint coffee also soothes the pain of difficult menstruation.

Mustard

Mustard has long been used as a medicine, but the seeds used to be ground and mixed with honey and vinegar then rolled into balls which could be stored for use as and when required...

The balls were then mixed with more honey or vinegar and this paste used as a poultice for all manner of aches and pains; it can be so used today provided that it is never placed directly on broken skin as, if it were, the rubbing action of the Mustard could delay the healing process ... it would also sting! Opera singers in the past always used Mustard balls to keep their lungs clear of congestion and improve their voices (Maybe some of today's 'pop' singers could do with some balls). They are also good for healing tooth and gum infections (the Mustard balls, not the 'pop' singers!)

Although Mustard is a powerful irritant and can cause blistering if applied directly to the skin, I have obtained great relief in applying mild table Mustard (ready mixed) directly from the jar or tube as an ointment in cases of frozen shoulder, stiff neck, chilled muscles and pleurisy.

To ease very bad cases of bronchitis, pneumonia and pleurisy, I also spread table Mustard on tissue handkerchiefs or babies napkin liners, which are then covered with a second layer of tissue, placed on the back or chest and covered with a hot-water bottle to make a very effective poultice without all of the messy preparation of hot cloths etc ... take care if sleeping with the poultice on to secure it well before settling down.

Once used as a medicinal snuff to cure the sinuses, Mustard powder seemed a cheap and handy medicine for me to use one day when my husband was suffering, so he was induced to take a hearty sniff ... after his eyes had stopped watering and his red nose had returned to normal, he stated that his head felt much clearer, so I know for a fact that this remedy does work ... but, be warned. . . this remedy should not be used shortly before going for a job interview or entering a glamour competition! Mustard is also an excellent spice herb for allaying the effects of rich or fatty meats, but I feel that there are so many varieties of Mustard available in the stores that it would be silly to take it in medicinal form for that purpose, when it is so easy to just take a little of your favourite Mustard with your meal as preventive medicine.

Although Mustard is so good for all these ailments, to my mind the most wonderful benefit it has is its ability to bring such fast and lasting relief to sufferers of those most dreadful of ailments, arthritis, rheumatism, sciatica and spondylitis. Sufferers of these complaints take heart, also take Mustard!

I have a jar of bath-powder in my bathroom which is made of a mixture of 1 teacupful of Mustard powder, 1 mugful of Epsom salts (commercial Epsom salts is best and can be obtained quite cheaply in the gardening departments of Boots or large stores). I strongly advise all sufferers to make themselves a jar and to use a handful of this in a hot bath at bedtime to ease the pain from any disease which affects tendons, muscles or joints.

Nutmeg

Nutmegs are exceptionally good, both as a medicine and as a valuable taste experience, so it is important to get the best. When buying whole Nutmegs always look for ones which are small and heavy, as the large light ones have had their essential oil commercially removed for medical use. . . as we are talking about Nutmegs as a medicine, that is the last thing we would want!

If using Nutmeg powder, always use a little more than you would if you were grinding it yourself to ensure its strength. Nutmeg oil, available in health-food stores and the like, is really too strong for day-to-day use which is what I advocate when using the contents of your spice shelf. However, if you are fortunate enough to have some of this very valuable oil, a few drops go a long way, so always use it diluted with olive, sunflower or almond oil in the ratio of 5 drops maximum of Nutmeg oil to every 1 tablespoonful of the base oil.

Nutmeg is an excellent tonic with nerve-relaxant properties so is very useful as a digestive aid, as our grandmothers knew well, hence their practice of sprinkling it over the milk pudding served after a heavy meal to induce an 'after-dinner-nap', which enabled the digestive processes to get well under way before any violent movements interfered with them (those of you who dislike the idea of strenuous exercise after a meal to 'work it off' take heart ... you are right ... a little rest is better!) A relaxing drink for sufferers of nervous tension, exhaustion or insomnia is simply made by grating a little Nutmeg onto a cup of hot milk and sweetening with honey ... Delicious Devonshire "Tatie Pie' is a good nutritious meal which can be easily made by lining a pie dish with thin shortcrust pastry, filling with alternative layers of thinly sliced potatoes, cream and grated Nutmeg and baking for 30-40 minutes in a moderate oven. This is excellent for children and invalids with weak stomachs and in fact, is enjoyed by everyone who tries it, making it a good standby as a 'non-medicine' help to health.

Sufferers of those most unglamorous complaints, piles and itching of the fundament, take heart ... and take Nutmeg ... its relaxant properties make this an excellent remedy for these embarrassing complaints ... especially if mixed with yogurt!

Believe me ... I would not joke over such a subject having been a sufferer myself in the past. Into a standard size pot of plain yogurt simply grate enough Nutmeg to cover the surface (about quarter of a teaspoon of dried, powdered Nutmeg is the equivalent amount), stir well and leave in the refrigerator for at least 24 hours before using as a cream to apply locally, after each visit to the toilet and after bathing ... If outer application does not appeal to you, relief will be obtained if a little of this mixture is eaten daily, last thing at night before retiring.
Of course, no advice on the use of Nutmeg is more universally used than that of carrying a whole Nutmeg about the person, whether it be in pocket, purse or coat lining (or, as one lady confessed in a whisper, up a knicker leg!) as a guard against, and ease for any pains caused by tension whether they be cramp, rheumatics or any other chronic nerve-directed pain ... it works!

Parsley

Parsley, the controversial herb which is only purported to grow for the woman of the house if she 'wears the trousers', is also her best friend if she has any ailments which owe their origin to her doing just that (or tights, or jeans!)

Very often it is the moist heat generated by our bodies which cannot evaporate if we wear tight clothing on our nether parts which gives rise to those dread complaints cystitis, thrush and vaginitis and a host of similar painful, irritating and embarrassing problems ... With Parsley on our spice shelf there is no need for anyone to suffer. .. what a statement, but quite true! Parsley cools the blood by regulating its acidity; this in turn soothes the nerve centres of the head and spine, in turn lowering blood pressure, expelling surplus fluid from the body tissues and acting as a natural antibiotic against infections. Speaking from many years of experience and with the hearty endorsement of many patients who have tried this remedy, one of the easiest ways of using

Parsley is simply to add 1 teaspoon of the dried herb to 1 large mugful of boiling water and stir several times during its cooling period, then strain into a screw-topped jar and keep in the refrigerator.

Use a little on a clean tissue as a rinse after each visit to the toilet, also moisten a sanitary pad with this and wear at night and, in extremely severe cases, dip a fresh tampon in the mixture before insertion to bring speedy and blessed relief. Gentlemen can obtain relief from similar 'taboo to mention' complaints by 'dipping into the jar' as and when required! Whether Parsley is fresh or dried in leaf or seed form, frozen, ready-rubbed, flaked or crisply-curled, its high mineral content and pleasant flavour must surely make it a most desirable herb to be found in as many homes as possible and I, for one, would consider the spice shelf poor that did not contain Parsley. Not only does it lend its flavour to a variety of savoury dishes such as sauces, soups, stuffings, rissoles, fish, mince etc., and to salads, cooked vegetables and dressings (not forgetting the rabbit pie which would not taste half as good without it), but it is also an invaluable remedy for home use as its action is never violent, yet it is very efficacious.

Parsley's reputation as a herb which 'helpeth men with weyke braynes to bayre drynke better' if taken beforehand, was probably what prompted the advice often given today never to drink alcohol on an empty stomach ... nothing changes does it? Parsley also has very strong deodorising properties and a bath with Parsley in it is said to invigorate the bather and captivate anyone coming in close proximity by their savour! I cannot vouch for the truth of that statement, but I can state that chewing a few Parsley seeds or drinking a cup of Parsley tea will subdue the strongest of mouth odours ... even that of Garlic!

Of course, the main benefit of Parsley must surely be its high iron and mineral content which, when Parsley is a regular addition to the diet, keeps the blood rich, alleviating anaemia and menstrual complaints. Its cooling action also fights all inflammation easing malaria, measles, fevers and flatulence!

Pepper

This is the unexpected hot remedy whose action is to cool the system ... you will be very surprised at the many benefits which can come to us as a result of simply taking more Pepper.

Although we take Pepper for granted as a cheap and readily available condiment, such was not always the case! When he was in his hey day, Atilla the Hun once demanded, and received, the enormous and then priceless amount of 3,000 lbs of Peppercorns as a ransom for the city of Rome ... it always seems a great pity to me that we do not value it as highly today (I am speaking of, black Pepper, as it is much more medicinal than white).

Black Pepper was always called Hoea Pepper in our home, as it is a very valuable remedy for complaints which end in 'hoea' for example diarrhoea, gonorrhoea, leucorrhoea etc. and, as it stimulates the tissues into acting for themselves instead of hanging around letting the rest of the body take their strain, it helps in cases of prolapsed bladder, rectum and womb. As it also destroys intestinal worms into the bargain, anyone would be foolish indeed who did not keep black Pepper on their table and use it as often as they like ... that's the best way to take it! Because of its action in regulating the blood pressure, it eases vertigo and nausea which so often are symptoms of irregularity in pressures. This also helps the body to detoxify itself and rid itself of fevers and disease caused by faulty elimination. Daily intake of black Pepper is said to help cases of paralysis of the tongue, so don't give any to a compulsive talker!

While on the subject of Pepper, I must of course mention the white Pepper which is on so many tables; this is made from Peppercorns which have had their piperine extracted by soaking, and then dried in the sun and crushed into the familiar powder.

Although it is no longer effective as a medicine for the various complaints already listed, if taken daily on food it is a very effective aid for those who suffer with habitual constipation. Its warming action is very beneficial to the digestive system and some instinct seems to tell us to take more Pepper with our meals when the digestion is upset ... do our bodies know best? Paprika or red Pepper is used more on the continent than here and is often called Hungarian Pepper due to its use in goulash and other spicy Hungarian dishes, in which it is delicious.

This is recognised by German herbalists as coming in three different grades, the most effective being a rich red colour,

while the brown and reddish yellow shades do not have much medicinal value. Due to its weak action and its risk of adulteration, it is used more often in veterinary treatments and is said to be effective in colouring the breasts of canaries with a beautiful red blush if given in their food (it also keeps the goldfish red to add a pinch to their water weekly!)
Personally, the best and most effective use that I have found for Paprika is to sprinkle it liberally on meals when anyone appears to be 'coming down' with a cold, sore throat or fever; it also eases sore throats if taken mixed with honey.

Rosemary

With its Latin name, Rosmarinus, meaning 'dew of the sea', with legend saying that it was a Rosemary bush that gave shelter to the Virgin Mary when she rested during her flight into Egypt, with its use in ancient days at betrothals, weddings, banquets, christenings and funerals alike, it is small wonder that this spice herb has retained its popularity and is one of the most commonly known herbs in use today as a food medicine.

Primarily, Rosemary is justly famous as the 'womens herb' due, no doubt, to its action on the bloodstream which quickly brings relief from all hormonal problems, including PMT, irregular and scant periods, hysterical depression and nervous complaints; it even lifts the terrible fatigue that comes at the menopause and brings so much unhappiness to sufferers, not least being the fact that so many women have partners who just do not understand how terrible it can be to cope with and that telling a sufferer to 'pull yourself together' causes even more pain.

There are many ways of taking Rosemary to relieve the symptoms of stress, even if they have been taking their toll of your health and strength of body, soul and spirit for many years (as is the case for thousands of sufferers all over the world). As this most wonderful of herbs can readily be obtained in tea bags I would suggest that the first move should be to obtain some and simply make as directed on the packet for instant and long-lasting relief.

However, as it is so versatile, always keep dried Rosemary on your spice shelf and use it daily.

One very tasty way of 'taking one's medicine' is to make some Rosemary wine, which is very simply done by adding 1 oz (or 25 gm) of dried Rosemary to 1 litre of sweet white wine and slowly bringing to the boil in a glass or enamel saucepan; set aside with the lid on for three days, after which time it is ready to strain and bottle and is ready for immediate use. This wine makes a welcome and very thoughtful present that need not cost much, yet is 'worth its weight in gold' to anyone who suffers from any of the following:

Spasmodic coughs, poor respiration, palpitations, headaches, nervous tension, depression, fatigue and water retention. It also stimulates the appetite, the kidneys and the whole nervous system. It is also said to revitalise the brain (so that's the reason for my mother telling me to take some!) and I know for a fact that a little of this Rosemary wine briskly rubbed into arthritic joints, paralysed limbs or gouty feet brings a great deal of relief and dabbing it on varicose veins brings bliss! This wine also makes a good first-aid antiseptic in case of emergency to apply to wounds, bites and stings, also whitlows and chilblains, but my personal view is that it is much too good to waste on such minor details!

For anyone who does not like to partake of the juice of the grape, a very good tonic with the same properties can be made by simply adding 1 teaspoon of Rosemary to the teapot or a good pinch to a cup of boiling water and sipping slowly whenever the need arises ... this can be sweetened with honey if desired and, added to the bathwater, is an excellent relaxant.

To make one of the very best hair tonics which will not only cleanse and tonify the scalp, clearing and preventing further recurrences of dandruff and similar problems, but will also settle the platelets of the hair, thus making it much more resistant to atmospheric pollution, and keeping it in good colour and gleaming with health, is very simple:

In a large glass or enamel saucepan put 1 oz (25 gm) of dried Rosemary, add 1 litre of spring water and bring to the boil and simmer on the lowest possible heat for about half an hour, stirring occasionally. Remove from the heat and allow to cool when, if stored in a tightly stoppered bottle it can be kept in the refrigerator and used as a scalp rub (simply apply at bedtime and rub well in, giving the scalp a good friction massage with the fingertips) or as a final rinse after washing (by adding one teacupful of the mixture to about 2 litres of lukewarm water and slowly pouring through the hair). This mixture is also a valuable aid against premature baldness and an excellent hair restorer when illness, shock or chemotherapy have caused temporary loss of hair ... what a wonder is Rosemary. This same mixture, when dabbed onto freckles or dark skin around the eyes or even the so-called 'liver spots' which come so often on the backs of our hands as we get older, will gradually lighten and tighten the skin so that regular use will soon have even young girls envying our beauty ... honestly!

Elizabeth of Hungary is reputed to have used Rosemary water to obtain her beautiful complexion which was not only famed all through the land, but got her a princely husband at 90 years old!

One of the beauties of Rosemary is that we do not have to take it medicinally to keep our health at the peak of perfection. We have all at some time experienced the taste sensation of spring lamb slowly steeped in Rosemary and served with little new potatoes, but have you tried adding Rosemary to other meat dishes to ensure that your body can deal with all crude meat tissues efficiently, thus aiding your digestion and giving yourself a rest from inner 'mechanical stress'? Do try it, you will find that some very tasty sauces which make a very welcome change from the 'norm' can be made using Rosemary, especially with the judicious use of lemon and garlic ... Mmmm! It can also be added to soups, stews, and savoury stuffings and even used as an instant 'cuppa-soup' by simply adding 1 thick pinch to a mugful of boiling water and adding a little sea salt and black Pepper to taste and drinking when cool enough, by which time the aroma should be irresistible!

I have often given this, poured over diced wholemeal bread or toast, as the first solid meal to patients suffering from any debilitating illness which has prevented them from eating for some time ... it is a very good appetite restorer.

I also find that very often the sick-room gets very 'stuffy' despite all our efforts to keep it fresh, and then 1 teaspoon of dried

Rosemary is worth its weight in gold ... try throwing 1 spoonful on the fire in a room where a bronchitic or asthmatic sufferer is resting, you will be amazed at the ease it will bring to their breathing ... or use a spoonful in some hot water to wash down walls etc., in the sick-room ... refreshing Rosemary!

Saffron

It is said that the first root of Saffron to be cultivated in the UK was smuggled out of the Levant in the hollowed-out head of a pilgrim's staff during the reign of Edward the Third (the pilgrim incidentally risking his life to do this) where it was planted at Saffron Walden, which gave the place its name.

At Saffron Walden, in the UK, it was proudly presented in silver cups by the Corporation to some of our Sovereigns and such was its value that the pound of Saffron which was presented to Queen Elizabeth the
First cost the princely sum of 5 guineas! Hardly surprising when you consider that the stamens of 40,000 flowers were required to make up this weight!
The reason for its worth was, I am sure, due to the fact that a little of this spice goes a long way and just to have a few stamens added to the cooking-pot or cake mixture ensured that the diner left the table with the certainty of having no after-

effects, other than a feeling of well-being. How many of us can say that today, I wonder, yet how easily we could with Saffron. In the West Country where I was born and bred, it is said that a little daily Saffron will prevent the taker from getting consumption and will bring the consumptive patient back from the dead, and for this reason Saffron cake is regularly served. As Saffron is still one of the most expensive spices, I only use it on special occasions or when absolutely necessary such as during nose bleeds when a few powdered stamens, sniffed into the nostril, will stop the bleeding almost immediately. A stamen rubbed on aching gums will anaesthetise them ... Super Saf!

Sage

Not for nothing did the ancients say that the man who took Sage daily would live for as long as he took it ... personally, I have experienced so many occasions in my life when I have thanked the Lord that there was Sage in my larder, that it would be almost impossible to list them all, but I will try.

First and foremost, of course, must come the fact that Sage is one of the best tonics available; its blood cleansing properties make it a genuine natural 'pick-me-up' and many is the time that members of my family would be 'one-degree-under' one minute and right as rain the next after taking no more medicine than a cup of Sage tea. For this we simply put one leaf of fresh, or a good pinch of dried Sage into a cup and add boiling water, stirring vigorously, then, when it cools to drinking temperature, just add honey to taste if desired and sip slowly ... this is extremely useful for all cases of fatigue whether of body, mind or spirit, no matter what the cause.

The addition of 1 tablespoonful of cider vinegar to this mixture turns it into a very well tested and tried remedy for coughs, colds, catarrh, etc., and has never yet been known to fail to bring relief.

It is especially effective as a mouthwash and gargle to ease the pain of and clear the body of toxins from quinsy, sore throats and tonsillitis, gingivitis, toothache and similar complaints; after gargling well and washing out the mouth, brush the teeth with this mixture to disinfect the area, it really is surprising how quickly this heals 'monster mouth'!

I will not insult your intelligence by presuming to give you any recommendations as to cooking with Sage, as it is one of the first savoury herbs we learn about, but I will remind you that a little
Sage added to any rich dish will ensure that pain and flatulence will not prevail at the end of the meal!

One Christmas when one of my daughters was only a few months old, she swallowed a tiny plastic duck (no doubt as a protest at not having the same festive fare as the rest of the family!) Father's exclamation of 'Blast me, that little old gal hev gone an ate that duck!' was merrily answered by my husband's shout of laughter and his comment 'better pass some Sage stuffing then and we'll soon get it back again!' And he was right, Sage went right to the spot and its cleansing action saved the day!

Another reason for my enthusiasm over Sage is that it soothes the nerves of the brain and it is surprising how often these nerves get inflamed causing feelings of pressure, 'crawling', giddiness, nausea, blurred vision, panic, stress and tension. Very often this leads to physical depression of the brain stem with its attendant boredom, apathy and sometimes even suicidal tendencies ... Now I am not saying that Sage alone can solve all of these problems but, with the help and understanding of your general practitioner and a little Sage tea taken daily, it is amazing how quickly life becomes worth living once again. Believe me, Sage tea can really be a God-send if you are in a situation of this kind ... I know because I have been there, and lived to tell the tale ... thanks to the saving grace of Sage.

The active principles of Sage make it more easily mixed with spirits than with water so for this reason (I kid you not!) it is usually to be found in this house in whole leaf form, steeping in a bottle of white wine (about a dozen leaves will be enough if you wish to try this remedy as it is very strong).

Sage wine has a very peculiar flavour but is unbeatable as an application for mouth ulcers and problems under the palate of dentures which can be extremely painful at times this is also good for easing the pains of teething but beware if your baby likes the medicine and is as intelligent as mine were, you could soon be spending more time tending to 'teething pains' than is strictly necessary ... ours lasted for nineteen years!

Sage wine also has such a strong antiseptic action that it has been known to clear up conditions which have resisted 'normal' medication for many years. This was proved to me very strongly when one of my youngsters brought home 'Old George', a gentleman of the road who had had dreadful leg ulcers since the war; Sage applied daily cleared them in six weeks, quite upsetting George!

As a medicine (leaving the best 'till last as usual), if taken in wineglassful doses daily it is still one of the best ways of easing pains in the joints caused by arthritis, rheumatism etc., also balancing the body fluids in cases of kidney or liver complaints, regulating and quickly dispelling the pains of menstruation, stopping lactation after childbirth and cleansing the stomach and intestines of all putrification where there are blockages or pockets, colitis, diverticulitis or other ulcerous or inflamed conditions ...

What a saviour is Sage.

Tarragon

Tarragon which we use as a piquant addition to salads, pickles and vinegars, was very highly thought of in the middle ages as a medicine when it was in constant use on the Continent, where its name Esdragon was the French translation of its Latin name Dranunculus or little dragon, due to its supposed power over all venomous beasts (including presumably the dragon!).

Be that as it may, I find it very handy to have some Tarragon vinegar in the house at jam-making time, as I have yet to find a better or more effective potion for dabbing on wasp stings and taking the sharpness out ... it is of course equally as good for any other stings and bites, but to my mind nothing is quite so terrible as a sting from the wearers of yellow and black suits! To make this very useful Tarragon vinegar, simply add half an ounce (or 12 gm) of dried Tarragon either in leaf, powdered or ready-rubbed form, to a bottle of cider vinegar or white vinegar and shake well, then allow to stand in a warm place for 24 hours before straining into a glass bottle with a good seal. Keep this on the front of your larder shelf to remind you that you now have not only a super sting-settler, but also an excellent condiment.

Called by the herbalists of old 'A friend to the head, heart and liver' it helps to restore the appetite, eases the pain of toothache, fights air-swallowing, flatulence and hiccoughs, and is very useful in the fight against obesity caused by fluid retention, yet all we have to do is use it as a table vinegar! What an easy medicine to take is Tarragon ... take it often, do.

Thyme

Now we come to the Master Herb ... I really could not have picked a better spice herb with which to end this book. .. although we use it often as an ingredient of the ubiquitous stuffing for a fowl or roast joint, most of the time we neglect to use this most versatile of herbs; never again I hope, after reading this book!

'Top to toe Thyme' is what my grandfather used to call this, healing as it does everything from bad breath to athlete's foot ... let me just give you a few simple tips to enable you to use Thyme as a healer in your home very easily and effectively.

Firstly, the dried Thyme that is sold in little tubs for pennies at the corner shop is going to be just as effective as expensively packaged and priced alternatives ... Thyme is Thyme.

As with any herb or spice, it is of course, more effective to use the fresh 'living medicine', so if you can grow a plant of Thyme either in your garden, window box or even in a pot on the kitchen window-sill, you will have the added advantages that not only will the enzyme action of the plant be very high, but you will also have an effective insect repellant close at hand. It is also a very good lift to jaded spirits to be able to squeeze a Thyme plant, releasing its delicious and uplifting aroma into the room and carrying its perfume with you on the palms of your hands ... this is Aromatherapy of which we hear so much recently, letting the aroma of your chosen herb medicine do the work of healing in a most pleasant and relaxing manner. What a pleasant and relaxing way of taking our medicine.

Every time we take a herb or spice scented bath we are giving ourselves an Aromatherapy treatment at home, and, if any of you suffer from acne, athlete's foot, skin complaints or any chest or lung problems, Thyme is the herb to use in this way. Simply put 1 teaspoonful of dried Thyme into a cotton handkerchief and tie tightly, then use this in the bath as a flannel, what could be more simple ... yet not much could be more effective! If anyone suffers from a very bad skin complaint which has resisted all the usual medications, it would be a good idea to make up a dozen or so bags at a time and keep them in the bathroom cupboard, using no other soap or cleansing agent on the skin at all but using the

Thyme bags night and morning until the problem has cleared, and clear it certainly will.

I used to make up several of these 'bathbags' and take them with us when the family went on holiday, as Thyme keeps the skin free from all those irritating itches and prickles that are so often the bane of the holiday. Also there is no better way of relieving sore and sweaty feet (after tramping over the moors all day following the 'locals' instructions as to how to find somewhere that is 'just half a mile down that lane' and walking about fifty miles in the process!) than to bathe them in a bowl of hot, fragrant Thyme water, and, if you decide to follow my example in this ... don't forget ... keep a bag for the first bath that you have when arriving home all tired, dusty and fractious after spending hours in traffic jams on the motorway or waiting for trains in dirty stations ... peace soon returns with Thyme.

Thyme tea, simply made by adding a cup of boiling water to about 1 teaspoon of the dried herb and seasoning or sweetening to taste (personally I add sea salt and paprika), is a very good tonic drink to take in the winter to keep the chest clear and ensure that chills do not develop into something bad. This tea, flavoured with a teaspoonful of lemon juice after rich or fatty meals, will soothe and ease the 'wambling' stomach and clear worms from the intestinal tract ... While on that subject, let me make it clear that most of the animal fibre that we eat carries small 'worms' called nematodes which are not destroyed by cooking and thrive best at the temperature of the human body; these worms cause all sorts of 'wandering symptoms' which have no apparent cause, baffling the sufferer and their practitioner alike ... There are only two medicines that I know of that are able to clear this situation, one is garlic and the other is Thyme, both of which, if taken regularly in our food, work well either together or separately to keep us in a state of perfect health ... Do please experiment in the kitchen and see how many ways there are to introduce either of these wonderful ingredients into the family fare; not only will you experience new and interesting tastes, but also know at the same time that you are helping yourself to health. Thyme tea also makes an excellent gargle and mouthwash that is very good at soothing sore gums and clearing bad breath, while for mastitis, Thyme tea can be applied as a hot poultice to ease the pain and reduce swelling while a 'cuppa-Thyme' soothes the inner turmoil that so often accompanies this complaint.

Charlemagne (that man again!) once ordered that Thyme must be grown in gardens; I wonder what would happen if the government made such a law today! It really would be a good idea, as this would take a great burden off the Health Services.

This beautiful fragrant herb should be treasured as if it was gold. One of the most effective tonic medicines available to man and worth its weight in gold can be easily made at home in this way:

Crush a whole head of garlic and mix with 1 oz (or 25 gm) of dried Thyme and stir into a jar of warmed clear honey. Keep in a warm place until required, stirring before use.

One spoonful of this mixture can be added to a cup of hot water and taken as required for any of the following complaints: arthritis, asthma, bronchitis, catarrh, colds, coughs (there is no better medicine in this world for whooping cough!), circulation problems including faulty blood pressure, cramps, digestive problems of all kinds, depression, energy loss, gout, influenza, kidney problems, neurasthenia, pleurisy, pneumonia, rheumatism, respiratory diseases, typhoid fever, tuberculosis and whitlows. The list seems endless and there are probably a hundred more ailments that can be helped by Thyme, but there is no more room in this book!

However, I will leave you with a little tip from my father which is 'When you are in doubt as to what course to take in life ... take Time. When you are in any doubt as to which medicine to take ... take Thyme.'

I hope that after reading this little book, you will help yourself to health not only with Thyme, but with the aid of all the healers on the spice shelf.